I0103887

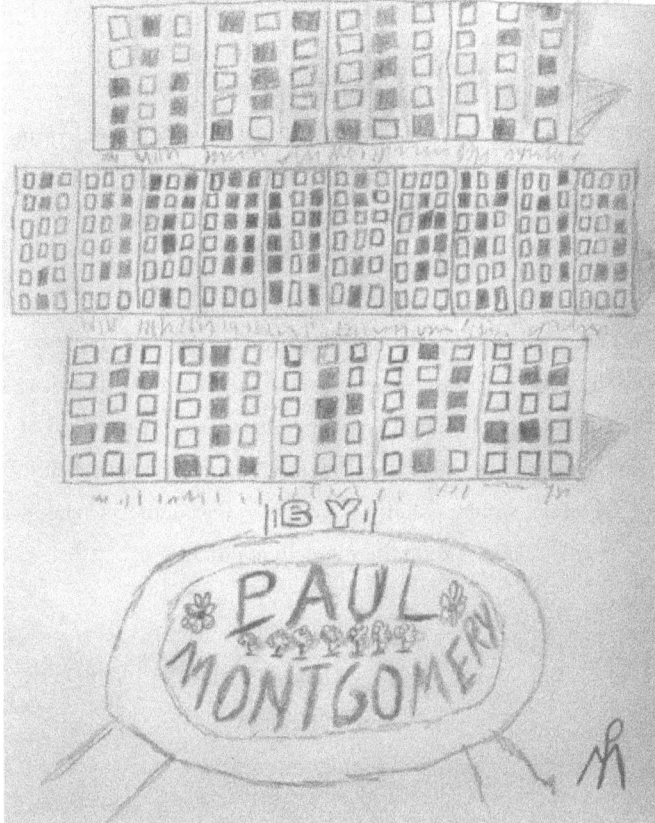

© Paul Montgomery 2011

All rights reserved. No part of this publication may be reproduced, stored in a retrieval system, or transmitted, in any form or by any means, electronic, mechanical, photocopying, recording, or otherwise, without the prior permission of Paul Montgomery or his heirs.

This book is sold subject to the condition that it shall not, by way of trade or otherwise, be lent, re-sold, hired out or otherwise circulated without the publisher's prior consent in any form of binding or cover other than that in which it is published and without a similar condition including this condition being imposed on the subsequent purchaser.

Cover art,
Frontispiece,
"Game of Health"
© Paul Montgomery 2011

ISBN 978-0-615-48398-6

First Edition

Googolplex Publishing

For the people

Table of Contents

Illustrations

Foreword

With the passage of healthcare reform you might think this book would be irrelevant. Things are so reformed now that your healthcare no longer sucks.

You would be wrong.

While healthcare reform did allow people to keep their child on their employer coverage until age 26 and thus made the section about full-time student status a snapshot of the horrors of yesteryear, the vast majority of the suckiness remains in tact. Because at each of the stages of your life that I examine you are ultimately led to conclude that....

8

Your Healthcare Sucks

Introduction

This book is directed to the majority of Americans who have employer-based health coverage. I am not going to address the quality of doctoring or nursing. This book is examining the nuts and bolts of actually getting the services to the people, in other words, administration.

As boring as an examination of administration may be, I feel I can make this worth your time. How about if I explain that the very health and life of you and your loved ones may depend on the information imparted in this book?

Hopefully, your situation never becomes that dire. And, frankly, most patients in emergent situations will be able to get the care they need in this country. However, I hope this book offers a soothing balm; that at least you are not alone in thinking that your healthcare sucks.

Rather, I write this book as an indictment of a crazy system that largely ignores the human being at its heart and as the reason for healthcare in the first place.

Birth and Childhood

There you are. Floating along in the amniotic sac without a care in the world. All your needs are provided by your mother.

But, soon enough you are thrust by the force of life into the sunshine and oxygen of our land-based, air-breathing world.

As you nestle in the loving arms of your parents, you count your blessings. You have been fortunate enough to be born into one of the greatest countries the world has ever known. You have all the advantages of the finest medical care of the 21st Century.

But, there is a hitch. You are really only entitled to the financial benefits of this miraculous system if your parents are sharp enough to get you enrolled. You're confident your folks will be able to sign you up for healthcare through your mommy or daddy's company.

———————————————————————

However, not everyone does sign their child up for benefits. Typically, there are restrictions related to the window in which to sign up for benefits. Often, this is 30 days.

I can hear the reader saying, "No one would be dumb enough to miss a 30-day window to sign up their child for health coverage."

I would say, "Yes! People do, indeed, miss their 30-day sign-up window. And, they are not dumb. These folks exist. I have spoken to them."

Becoming a parent for the first time is an extremely stressful time. Oftentimes, signing up for medical benefits is the last thing you think about. Perversely, this is sometimes caused by the very health of your child. In other words, parents of an exceedingly ill child may be so busy caring for their child that they forget to contact their benefits administrator to sign up their children for medical insurance. From my experience, this is true. Sad, but true. I have spoken to these people.

(Note: I will be drawing from my own personal experience in describing how your healthcare sucks. Some of these instances will seem too unrealistic to have happened. Take the above example. I can hear some very sensible people saying, "This is ridiculous. These people know they have a sick child. Of course, they are going to sign up the child for benefits."

I would answer back, "Have you ever had a sick child? If you did, you would realize how all-encompassing their care becomes. Taking care of the immediate physical needs of your child overwhelms any petty bureaucratic requirement to contact your benefits administrator."

Montgomery's Axiom

Having to meet a petty bureaucratic requirement will ensure that some people do not meet the same.

"So there! Dispute that!")

Maybe a little about my own background is needed here. I work for a company; if it was around in 1002, it would have been called BDR. So, at BDR I work as a benefits specialist. I'm the person you call on the phone when you need to sign up your child for your employer-based health benefits. I work for clients that are household names and members of the Fortune 500 or are major local government entities.

One of the ironies of my life is that I work administering the human resources benefits of these major employers yet BDR treats it employees like shit. Today, we are hosting a visit from a major U.S. passenger rail company. I imagine they are considering using our services.

In anticipation of their visits we started receiving little enhancements to our environment. All of the specialists and representatives received new nameplates and framed diplomas of our training accomplishments. Mine was wrong, as it only contained one of my disciplines. I am trained in Health and Welfare, Defined Contribution, Defined Benefits, and Payroll plans. Mine only said, "Health and Welfare".

Also, we got new furniture for our lobby and 2nd floor landing. The day the furniture arrived an E-mail was sent from the site manager that we, the employees, should not sit in the furniture in the lobby. That we were to use the furniture in the break rooms only. Our crusty butts were not welcome in the new leather and fabric. Everyone knows that you don't let the slaves into the parlor.

On my way out the door that day I saw the site manager sitting in the lobby with a smile on her face. We also got some plastic plants in the bathrooms.

———————————————————

You didn't have the good fortune to be born in our fine country. But, a loving couple has decided to take you into their hearts and arms and bring you to this country.

Yes, you are being adopted and you just know these great people are going to be wonderful parents. You also know that they will help take care of your medical attention.

———————————————————

Ah, here is where the hitch appears. Some companies are sticklers in demanding that the adoption be finalized before the child can qualify for the company's insurance.

Sometimes, parents have physical custody of the child before an adoption. Sometimes, no adoption is in the works.

A grandparent may take in a grandchild for any number of reasons. These relationships can be formalized with a guardianship, or not.

Companies vary in their requirements for dependent eligibility. Some require a formal, legal relationship. Some simply request your statement on a recorded phone line or via a secure website that you provide a majority of support for the child or that you and the child are in a parent-child relationship. Some entities just require the child be your legal child with no exception.

This can result in the cruel situation that two children in the same house with the same ostensible parents can have very different healthcare situations, one child covered with the parents in their group insurance and the other requiring individual* coverage or going without.

Someone may argue, "Isn't there the Children's Health Insurance Program from the federal government? This should get those children covered."

I would answer, "That may be the case in theory, but then why am I having these parents call to try and get children covered."

---

* Individual coverage means getting coverage yourself, as opposed to, the group coverage or employer-based coverage I've been describing.

Perhaps, a little more background on me will help. Yesterday, there was a rumor of more layoffs. We've been having successive rounds of layoffs this year.

The first round took out a layer of management and higher-paid staffers. Mostly, it was as though a line was drawn at a certain salary level. If your head was above that line it was chopped off. There were exceptions, of course.

Many of the workers fired had been with the company for years. They had survived a few mergers and takeovers. Their salaries were legacies of better times.

About eight years before, when the call center was just getting started and was being run by a company I'll call Cantaloupe, perks were good and employees were making a decent wage. They had free lunches and snacks. Employees were encouraged to take a break after a bad call.

Employees who had survived from this time got a wistful look in their eye as they described the circumstances of their employment. At that time, human resources outsourcing was relatively new and there was a drive to recruit and retain good quality workers. There was little competition so wages could be high.

Even with higher wages and perks, the economies of scale and technological advances of call management and centralized knowledge databases allowed human resources outsourcing companies to create decent jobs that probably paid less in wages and pension, yes, pension, benefits than prior human resources jobs but that were generally good and rewarding.

Now, the high wages are gone, the pensions are gone, the perks are gone, the 401(k) match was suspended, and sometimes, the jobs themselves are gone. All of this leaves us at work awaiting more layoffs today.

———————————

You've survived your childhood and are now moving to young adulthood. You are off to college, hopefully, and a new job. You are probably going to get married.

To keep your healthcare you've got to avoid some pitfalls. You've got to think about retaining your dependent eligibility.

What if you drop out or get married precipitously or have to take full-time employment to finance your education? You may find you've lost your insurance. And, if Mom or Dad forget to report it in time, you've lost your chance for COBRA coverage.

COBRA coverage is a funny beast. COBRA itself stands for Consolidated Omnibus Budget Reconciliation Act. Basically it allows you to retain group coverage after the loss of eligibility.

The cost of COBRA coverage is 102% of the cost of your current coverage. This sounds pretty reasonable, but when you consider the 100% is made up of the employee portion and the usually unseen employer portion, COBRA coverage can seem shockingly expensive.

Especially, when you consider that COBRA was designed in the 1980's when coverage was less expensive and before the last decade's 131% inflation in healthcare costs. The last 2% is an administrative fee, this being paid to a third-party administrator who takes on the duty of signing you up for benefits and taking payments.

But, enough about COBRA, I've got to discuss this last little bit about your diminishing dependent eligibility. As you've probably guessed by now, every company and entity is different in the way they determine aging out of dependent eligibility.

Some will allow you to continue for a few years past 18 or 19 as long as you are a full-time student, generally carrying 12 credits at a college, etc. The permutations on who is or isn't a full-time student can be mind-boggling. For instance: what about summer break, beauty school, schools using the quarter system, non-traditional schools that don't assign credits, when you are enrolled, when you begin, when you return? What if you are: on leave, sick, in the military, pregnant, fail a course, accepted but not enrolled?

What if you have to drop out of school as a result of an illness? Does this mean you lose your healthcare? When does your coverage actually begin? When you enroll? When you are accepted? When you begin classes? It's better not to slice that sausage too thin.

As a call center representative it is my job to get the person who is asking those all-too-logical questions off the phone as soon as possible. There are no good answers to those questions. The plan rules aren't that specific.

Nobody ever laid out the exact jagged borderline between being covered and not being covered in situations where your full-time student status is in doubt. This can lead to the disconcerting questions and non-answers raised above.

Often, the layout of this imaginary land is drawn by a benefits administrator. Your inclusion or expulsion is at their whim.

———————————————

You've stopped being a full-time student, or perhaps you never were. You have reached the age where your eligibility for your parent's group coverage ends. You may be 19, 23, 25, or 26 depending on the particulars of the plan.

Hopefully, your parent remembers to call in and have you removed from coverage in a timely fashion so you can get COBRA coverage. Because aging out is based on your date of birth in our database it is a relatively automatic process. But, mistakes do happen.

More likely, you've stopped meeting eligibility requirements in one of three major ways: you've moved out on your own, gotten married, or now have a job with insurance. You'll notice only one of those events actually provides you with new coverage. Otherwise, you will need to rely on COBRA and its 36-months length as a result of a loss of eligibility.

You'll get a COBRA package 14 days
after the COBRA benefits administrator is
notified of your termination. You'll have 60
days to decide whether or not to take
COBRA. COBRA will become effective the
date of your coverage loss so you will not
have a gap in coverage.

———————————————————————————

Welcome to adulthood.

Adulthood

You are starting your first job with health benefits. You are looking forward to being a responsible adult, getting married, buying a house, starting a family.

As a new hire you have a certain 30-day window to make your benefit elections. You may have a waiting period to go through before your benefits begin.

If you miss your 30-day window you may have to wait until the next open enrollment period. This is typically in the fall for the coming new year.

Some companies or entities may

require you to have health coverage. The default setting for your new hire election may be some pre-chosen health plan rather than having no coverage. So, even if you miss the deadline for your elections you will have *some* health insurance.

A few of the new hires will call all confused after their enrollment period, sometimes years after, and think they have health coverage. They thought it was automatic.

They will insist. Then, you will ask them if they received their new hire enrollment materials. No or maybe not. It was so long ago. Then, you will ask them if they have been having deductions for their medical. At this point they may feign ignorance or actually be ignorant to the idea that health coverage actually costs money.

Most of the time this is simply a case of getting them signed up during the next open enrollment period or with a qualifying life event. They would have to pay out-of-pocket for their medical care until we can get them signed up for insurance.

Many of these non-insureds are young and are taking the gamble that they won't need insurance. Some really are ignorant of such things and simply let enrollment slide.

The truly unfortunate occurs when they actually need insurance and lots of it; only to find that it is not available now but in a few months. Or, how about needing coverage for their child. Sometimes, they think the child was signed up by some magical means. No, you actually have to tell us you have a child who needs coverage.

———————————

You have met a wonderful person and are getting married next Saturday. You know you can sign up your spouse for health coverage with your company.

You are so eager; you call to add her before the wedding and are told you need to wait until the marriage actually occurs.

They cannot take future life events you are told. You can call after the wedding and you have a 30-day window to add her to your coverage.

———————————

Adding a new spouse to your coverage seems straightforward enough. Get hitched; add your spouse.

Think again. This area is as complex

and as rife with pitfalls as that morass, full-time student status, for instance: domestic partnerships, common-law marriages, same-sex spouses.

Let's start with domestic partnerships. What does this mean? This is human resource speak for a marriage by non-legal means. The interpretation of domestic partnership is up to each individual company.

Companies try to be fair-minded in their definition of domestic partnership. This fair-mindedness varies as companies vary. Some companies, recognizing that gay marriage is largely unavailable, make domestic partnerships available for same-sex couples only. This is seen as a fair counterbalance to heterosexual marriage.

Other companies think the way to be fair is to allow any couple, gay or straight, to have a domestic partnership. That way, the company does not have to delve into your sexual orientation.

Some states allow and other states recognize common-law marriages. States that recognize common-law marriage do not allow such to occur but will acknowledge them when the couple moves from a state allowing them.

The laws surrounding common-law marriage vary from state to state, also, from company to company. Some companies require nothing but your statement of marriage. Whereas, some will need documentation, a common-law marriage certificate.

Marriage really seems to engender feelings of discrimination. Gay folks get upset that they are unable to marry. (They are in some jurisdictions of late.) Straight people get mad when special arrangements like domestic partnerships are created for same-sex-only arrangements.

Out of companies' desire to be fair, come only half measures that satisfy some while leaving others hurt. Let me give an example, a same-sex domestic partnership of six-months duration allows the coverage of the partner, such a similar heterosexual arrangement would leave the partner uncovered. Conversely, a gay partnership of six-years duration leaves one partner uncovered as the company does not recognize domestic partnerships while a similar common-law arrangement among heterosexuals allows partner coverage.

At the workplace, the rumored layoffs did not materialize. But, I've been thinking of some of the folks I know there and how I have not seen them in several months. There was H.C. He helped interview me.

He worked in the quality assurance department. Most of the folks in that area were fired in the first two rounds of layoffs.

You'd think with all those quality people gone, that BDR doesn't have a commitment to quality. Other employees have taken on their duties.

Most of the trainers were fired, too. The quality assurance people and trainers were better compensated. Remember that imaginary line I was talking about earlier. Their salaries were probably above that imaginary line.

A time or two I was invited to apply for a position as a quality assurer or a trainer. I'm glad now that I demurred.

My interest did not lie in either of those directions, even though it would have meant being off of the phone. And, when business turns down those further from the customer are the first to be cut.

———————

You are entering the yearly open enrollment period for your company. Mostly this occurs in the fall of the year for coverage in the coming year.

Now, you can add any dependents you want who are eligible. You can change your insurance carrier. Basically, you need to make a new decision on the coverage available to you.

———————————————

This sounds pretty straightforward. But, there are pitfalls. For example, your spouse's coverage may have a different open enrollment period that needs to be coordinated with yours.

Also, open enrollment appearances can be deceiving. The cost of your coverage may have remained the same, so you assume it has not changed. However, your out-of-pocket maximum and deductible may have increased. Your service co-pays may have increased. Your covered benefits may have decreased.

Even when your premiums increase, don't assume the benefits have stayed the same. You may be subject to the same diminution of benefits while seeing your premiums jump.

At this point in the narrative I think I

should write about my own health dilemma. In this age of confession, there is often mentioned the healing benefit of sharing your misery.

I am nearing the six-year anniversary of a fungal ailment. At least, it is my assumption it is fungal in nature. It has never been properly diagnosed.

In fact, the last doctor I saw said he did not see I had anything wrong with me. (This didn't stop him from prescribing medication and asking me to schedule a follow-up visit.) So, dear reader, you may have the luxury of thinking I have some psychological malady. For me, I must continue on the assumption I am suffering with my undiagnosed illness.

Way back in 1982 I suffered from ringworm. That is what I think my present fungus is. Although I can't remember the particulars, it seemed like I was completely cured in about a week. I was in New Zealand at the time.

They have nationalized healthcare; and while I can't credit this with the rapidity of the cure, it seems like they had me diagnosed and on the mend in one visit.

I recently made an appointment to see my eighth doctor/physician's assistant in my current case. Now, at the beginning of this story I said I wasn't going to beggar the nation's doctoring. I think, in general, it is fine. In my particular case, it sucks.

———————————————————

You decide to move. You have found a lovely affordable house for you and your beautiful spouse to move into.

After you move, you call your friendly benefits specialist who informs you that due to your move to a new zip code you will no longer be eligible for your present HMO.

———————————————————

HMO's are, what are known as, zip code-driven. This means if you move to an area with a new zip code, sometimes even across the street, you will have to pick a new insurer as the HMO is simply not available.

This makes it worth your while to investigate your zip code/HMO situation. Some people will try to twist their address into knots so they can be in the HMO service area.

One tale is worth telling. A lady moves but does not report it immediately to her human resources department. When she does report it six months later, she is automatically moved to a PPO (Preferred Provider Organization) retroactive to the move date. She has totally missed her 30-day window to make her election.

Any procedures she had done in that six-month timeframe will have to be resubmitted to her new carrier. She would then have to wait for open enrollment to roll around to find a plan more to her liking.

This is not at all an unusual scenario. Just yesterday, I had a similar case. She had gone on leave and when she needed to pay for coverage via direct billing she had let it lapse. That meant her HMO coverage stopped.

When she returned to work she was automatically elected into a PPO as she did not make a new selection. She had continued to go to the HMO — oftentimes there is a time lag between cancellation and notification going to the carrier. So, any care she had received in the HMO would need to be resubmitted to the PPO for coverage.

This makes me think of another call I received yesterday. It is slightly off the topic but it does display some folk's mentality.

The caller was inquiring about his healthcare flexible spending account. This allows you to set aside pre-tax dollars and then submit claims for reimbursement. You can have co-pays, prescriptions, deductibles, and other expenses reimbursed.

Typically, this account resets to zero every year. For example, if you elected $1000 in 2010, in 2011 it would revert to $0 unless you actively elected another amount. Also, if you have an unclaimed balance in the account, you lose it.

This fellow was wondering where the money in his flexible spending account was. He called the plan administrator and they told him he had not participated since 1988. 1988! Yes, 21 years before.

I assured him that you needed to make an election every year. I went as far back as January of 2007 in researching that he had not participated since at least that date.

Forgetting to report a life event for six months or a year-and-a-half is not at all unusual. Any call center representative who is reading this will be nodding their head in agreement. You know you are.

Your wonderful daughter is leaving for college. You've already notified your benefits specialist of her full-time student status. Whew!

However, you later find that your daughter is only covered by your HMO in case of emergency. Routine doctor visits are no longer covered as she is no longer in the coverage area.

This kind of situation happens all the time and in many permutations. Wife moves before husband, husband moves before his family. The employee is on a temporary assignment.

Some companies try to accommodate this situation more than others. Some allow you to have two different kinds of coverage, either for the student or the family members who are out of the HMO area.

Some entities make no accommodation whatsoever. If your child leaves for an out-of-area college and you have an HMO, you will have to wait until open enrollment to change to a PPO plan. You may have only one official address. If one of your family moves they will simply have to wait until you change your address or plan.

This inflexibility reminds me of our vacation policy at BDR. I recently put in for an afternoon off. This was denied. It was no big deal because the evening kickoff of the dance film festival I wanted to attend did not begin until 8:00 pm.

Anyway, my time-off request was denied for a reason that I surmise had something to do with the 8% rule referred to in a forwarded E-mail I received. I don't know what the 8% rule refers to. Workload? Lack of vacation time? Too early in the fiscal year? I guess if I cared more I would inquire. Also, I don't want to give the impression of a troublemaker in these economic hard times. Especially since I don't need the time off.

At BDR all vacation time expires with the end of the fiscal year on June 30th. This is exceedingly annoying, infuriating even.

In theory, you could take a vacation anytime of the year. But, because typically you earn vacation time as the year proceeds, you start the fiscal year with a zero balance. Again, in theory you could go into the negative one week. I don't know about such things in actual practice.

The two people I know who took vacations in July, did so without pay. Yes, time off without pay for a vacation in July.

So, because everybody is building up a vacation balance that they have to use by June 30th, everyone tries to take time off in June. Eventually, this starts to eat into the minimum number of call center representatives needed. Then, you guessed it, vacations have to be denied.

My first year with the company I had to forfeit a couple of days of vacation. By the time I actually started to earn vacation it was April. When I got around to asking to use my time off there was only one day available to me in the middle of the week. I had a really great Wednesday vacation.

To this day, if you want to set a representative off, start talking about vacation. People will grit their teeth, their eyes will flair, voices will raise. Best to not even bring up the subject.

By the by, I was able to leave a little early that Friday (the start of the dance film festival), if only to avoid overtime. You see, I had worked extra hours earlier in the week.

You think I might have had the choice of leaving early or taking the overtime, as I could use the money and I had given the company time when they needed it. Instead, it was presented as something I did not have a choice in.

Again, this is not the moment in time to cause unnecessary trouble. I had asked for the vacation time previously and it had not been granted, so I might as well take the time off.

Typically, in such situations where you leave work early you can use vacation time so you don't miss work hours. If I had been able to use vacation hours, then I would still have received the pay for my extra hours, albeit not at an overtime rate.

I hinted at using vacation hours and was denied most likely because BDR is trying to prevent paying for the extra hours of overtime. This was still all right with me as I am trying to save vacation time until Christmas so I can take my daughter with me to visit her grandmother.

I swear I will get back to your healthcare in a moment, but bear with me for a few more paragraphs. I thought of a couple of things I need to express.

The person I was having my vacation, overtime, time-off inquiry with was my immediate manager. She is an all right person and I like her. I just thought I would share some vignettes of her and some other characters at BDR.

My manager was watching the Michael Jackson memorial at work the other day. She and the technical analyst for my team were both watching and comparing notes. How good Jennifer Hudson was, etc. Yes, the Internet allows you to watch TV at work.

I don't want to make myself seem blameless in all the Internet usage. You will find me surfing relentlessly between calls. I almost never watch video though, as that sucks a lot of bandwidth and I find having to use headphones would be too much of a giveaway. Other employees do not feel so compelled and enjoy music and moving pictures from their computer monitors.

The nature of the call center business is feast or famine. Mondays are atrocious with calls coming back-to-back at certain times of the year or the month. Fridays are the opposite end of the spectrum with whole hours going by uninterrupted. This slack time allows for leisurely reading of horoscopes or newspapers.

I just had a chilling thought. The I.T.

people are increasingly making parts of the Internet inaccessible. E-mail and social networking websites are no longer available. How soon before access to astrological websites gets shut down? The funny part is that the younger, more technically-minded staffers can still access verboten websites while us oldsters are limited to the news.

Your spouse gets a new job that offers better medical benefits. This would allow you a new 30-day window to drop her and yourself from your medical benefits.

Since your dental is better with your company, you and she can stay on your dental and other benefits.

This all seems very straightforward and for the most part it is. One exception to this is if your spouse goes to work for the same company. Then, typically the company has rules and prohibitions against what is called dual or double coverage.

The rules against double coverage prohibit a person from having their spouse as a dependent and the spouse having their own primary coverage as an employee. What happens in this situation is that the husband and wife will get the employee's health plan that is cheapest with the most benefits.

This brings up the interesting fact that within one company there will be many different health plans that vary in terms of company contributions and the employee's share. The main differences are between management and labor, non-union and union, and the workers of one particular factory or geographic area and another.

The employees with the most generous healthcare terms tend to be management and unionized labor. The differences in factories or geographic areas usually relate to rates of unionization, legacy plans from takeovers and mergers, or the availability of a particular HMO or PPO.

A slight bureaucratic headache can occur when a person tries to sign up for health coverage at the same company her spouse works for. She first has to have her spouse drop her from coverage before the computerized benefit database will allow her to be added on her own. The computer having been programmed to prevent dual coverage.

I don't want to give you the impression

the life of a call center representative is all bad. There can be great joys to the work. For example, trying to help someone who is all confused and you make sense of their situation and you encourage them to take action to protect their benefits. These moments are very rewarding and help you to have pride in your job. You absolutely need them to help you get through the troublesome or frustrating calls.

Just the other day I was speaking to a new father who had missed the 30-day window to add his newborn to coverage. He swore up-and-down that he had added his child. He had called the benefits center, he said. He had talked to a benefits specialist. They told him his child was added to his benefits.

On reviewing his account information we did not show that he had called the benefits center. We did not show that he had added his child to his healthcare.

He was offered the appeal process. This process can take as long as 180 days to resolve.

By the time he called me, I was the fourth benefits specialist he had spoken to that day. People will often call back to try and get a different answer, or because they did not trust the information they received. And, sometimes, a benefits specialist can make a mistake. We are human, after all.

The three previous benefits specialists had given him the same information; that he had missed the 30-day window to add his child and that he would need to file an appeal.

This new father was not taking the news well. He was very upset. Of course, he said, one of us could make an exception for him and add the child to coverage.

I explained, as I am sure the other benefits specialists had, that we had to abide by the plan rules, that we did not show the child having been added, that to add the child to coverage now he would need to file an appeal.

Eventually, he asked to speak with a supervisor. I scheduled a supervisor callback for the next day. I also assured him the supervisor would provide him the same information.

Contrast this situation with a similar situation involving a newborn child. When a parent calls to add a baby to coverage they do not have a Social Security number. We take the information for the child and ask them to call back when they get the Social Security number.

These parents will sometimes call back in two or three weeks. Their children have been assigned Social Security numbers for accounts they will not be paying into for at least a decade.

And, I believe that whenever you call the Social Security Administration they will assign your child a Social Security number. It does not matter if you wait one or two months or one or two years or one or two decades. They will assign your child a Social Security number and that is all there is to it. Your child is set up for disability and retirement benefits, potentially a half to two-thirds of a century in the future.

━━━━━━━━━━━━━━━━━━

You need to take some leave from your job. You are going to school or completing a military assignment.

Your boss says to call and get information about your health coverage.

━━━━━━━━━━━━━━━━━━

The rules on leave are all across the

board between employers. Most typically you are going to find that your coverages as an active employee end with the start of your leave. You will typically be offered COBRA coverage.

If you are no longer going to receive a paycheck as an employee, then paying for COBRA coverage can be a difficulty. In the military you will probably be covered by their healthcare. As a student you can hope that the school has a good and cheap health service.

You are going on leave but this time it is because you are about to become a new parent.

You are going to take as much time off work as you can to enjoy your new child.

Again, here the problem is continuing your coverage. Can you maintain your coverage and at what rate? Are you allowed to keep your active coverage at an employee rate while you take care of your child?

This gets into issues of leave, such as

whether it is paid or unpaid, family leave. Of course, California is different in having its own type of paid leave so new parents can bond with their child.

Yesterday ended tough for me. I had a couple of difficult calls back-to-back. Without going into specifics, the first I mishandled by thinking I knew best when I didn't. The misapplication of a usually successful technique to the wrong situation.

The second was a lady who was taking a disability retirement and was sitting with her lawyer as she called. She and the lawyer wanted to question everything. It felt like I was on the stand for a half hour.

Not that I blame either of the participants. They were both trying their best to obtain their healthcare. And, I try to analyze the tough calls so I can improve my performance.

I hate disability calls. Basically, I have very little information to provide them. The information in the knowledge base I use at work covers disability in a cursory manner.

The disabled people, too, are either very sad, depressed, or hostile. For the most part it seems like they get screwed from every angle by any company they work for.

The disabled folk are extremely knowledgeable about their benefits. These are folks who have nothing but time to study the plan documents.

And, the way our workforces handle disability it quickly becomes adversarial. As soon as someone becomes disabled, they hire a lawyer. On the company side they try and protect themselves both from fraud and legitimate expenses. Any loophole or way to deny your benefits as a disabled person will be used against you.

Take my advice, DO NOT become disabled.

Is it foolish of me to believe that there should be a better way? One in which a person would be guaranteed healthcare whether they were disabled or not? How about, especially if they were disabled?

Some of the perversity of our current system actually rewards the denial of healthcare to the disabled. If, a company can avoid a disabled person's expenses, it has sewn up a hole in its bottom line. And, most companies continue to charge for insurance coverage from the meager disability pay.

Even writing about this I find myself getting angry and sad...

I had to take a break and come back to this after I had calmed those feelings.

You wake up in a hospital. You had an accident at work. Who knows when you will return to work, if ever?

You put aside thoughts of your ailments. You call a lawyer and look ahead as you prepare yourself for conflict. You know that you may have to fight, possibly for the rest of your life, and you make yourself strong for the struggle.

One lonesome little sideroad of how your healthcare sucks is the worker's compensation area. Even as your employer may be subsidizing your healthcare, it is a paradox that this same healthcare will not cover workplace injuries.

Workplace injuries are paid for by worker's compensation insurance. Worker's compensation grew out of the need to take care of workers and hold employers responsible for the health and safety of their workers. This is a form of insurance that employers are required to provide and is often administered by the state government. This is mostly because the insurance companies can make no profits from this area and gradually the state took over the responsibility for this worker's insurance.

I am no expert on worker's compensation. I apologize for any major discrepancies to this pencil sketch of worker's comp. I just wanted to show how yet another form of insurance affects your coverage. The worker's compensation arena is enough of a mess without having me dive into its problems.

But, this is a good example of how your healthcare sucks. You're cruising along thinking you've got one kind of insurance when suddenly you are plunged into another insurance world that has its own arcane rules that you basically know nothing about. And, you are best off consulting a lawyer even before a doctor.

You are losing your job. You are being fired, terminated, laid-off, let go, reduced, rationalized, right-sized, leaned and meaned, canned, sacked, shown the door, axed, termed, 86'ed, given the pink slip.

You know there is something called

COBRA that would allow you to continue your coverage. You don't really know how it works but it provides some comfort that you can continue to cover yourself and your family.

————————

COBRA sounds like a snake. It brings to mind the winding serpent of the caduceus. Actually, COBRA is an acronym for the Consolidated Omnibus Budget Reconciliation Act of 1985.

COBRA coverage allows you to continue the coverage you and your family had while you were an active employee. The cost of COBRA is 102% of the cost of your active coverage.

On the surface, the cost seems reasonable. It is when you break down the cost that the coverage can seem out of reach. The 100% of the 102% is 100% of the active cost including both the employee and employer contributions.

If your employer pays 75% of the cost of your active coverage, COBRA coverage would represent a four-fold increase in your cost. If your employer pays 50% of your active costs, COBRA represents a doubling of your costs.

The 2% of COBRA's 102% is an administrative fee. This is charged by the new administrator. COBRA is often overseen by a third-party administrator.

The silly thing is that you see this increase when you have lost your job and can least afford a cost increase. So, from meager unemployment insurance you have to make up this rise in your healthcare costs.

As it stands now there is a federal subsidy of 65% of the cost of COBRA coverage for those who have lost their jobs as a result of the current recession. Not only is this a massive subsidy of the health insurance industry, one of the most profitable industries, but it seems to me a massive admission that COBRA as it stands now is a failure.

Not only the cost of COBRA is a disaster but typically the service you get suffers as a result. Instead of one benefits administrator you typically have two. Let me tell you that two benefits administrators are not better than one.

Just a quick aside before I continue on with any COBRA discussion. I hear opponents of single-payer healthcare rant about having a bureaucrat between you and your doctor. That makes me laugh. What do you think I am? I am a bureaucrat. I am between you and your doctor right now.

People call in and they want healthcare coverage for themselves or their family. Based on plan rules I have to deny this to them. A large part of my job is telling people, "No!"

There are polite ways to do so and BDR always wants us to try to use what they call "positive positioning". In other words, don't say "No!"

Don't tell a participant that they missed their 30-day enrollment window as a new hire and they and their family will have to wait for open enrollment for employer group healthcare coverage. Tell them they have a chance to purchase individual insurance on the free and open market for themselves and their family until January of next year.

I am being a tad facetious here. It is hard. What would you say?

Anyway, back to COBRA, the morass that is COBRA. Usually, your new COBRA administrator will send you paperwork, take your elections, and your payments. For actual sending of your information to the insurance carriers they will usually rely on your current benefits administrator, BDR.

This means that when there is a problem with your insurance carrier not having your information, you can get batted around between your COBRA and benefits administrator. One blames the other and transfers you in turn.

There is something funny in call center work. There tends to be a lot of blaming the other person.

When you get a call transferred from payroll, those payroll jerks didn't do their job. When it's from health and welfare, those people are so lazy. I'll have to help this person because everyone in this call center is sitting on their hands and I'm the only one who actually cares about the participants.

This leads back in a circular fashion to the transferring I was speaking about for COBRA. To sign-up you use the COBRA administrator. For your data to actually get transferred to the insurance carrier you need to speak with BDR. When something fouls up and the carrier does not get your information, you will be batted between the two and your representative will always be convinced it is the other side that is causing your angst.

How to Commit Insurance Fraud

Let's say you are an unethical COBRA administrator. All those funds coming through your door are awfully tempting. And, to paraphrase one U.S. Senator, insurance companies seem to regard fraud as a normal course of business. I'm picking on COBRA here but really this could apply to many companies and situations.

If you take a small fraction of your COBRA participants and never forward the money to purchase insurance, it is virtually undetectable. Let's say ½ of 1% of all monthly COBRA participants are kicked off of coverage because COBRA does not forward their premiums. Over the course of a year you have pocketed 6% of member premiums.

This is not an ideal system. A certain percentage of your customers will call and complain. They will have tried to see a doctor and discovered their coverage was cancelled. So, these customers will engage in the verbal ping-pong of trying to get their coverage reinstated between yourself and BDR. Enough people will call and complain that you will not be able to realize 6% profits.

Let's say 20% of the people so cancelled will get their coverage reinstated.

This puts your gain somewhere south of 5%. This is all to the good.

As long as the number of people so cancelled remains under 5%, their impact is statistically insignificant. A common assumption with statistical sampling is that 95% is as close as needed to 100% to provide confidence in your results. In other words, the 5% of people cancelled do not outweigh the 95% of people covered.

The 20% of the cancelled who become aware of their situation do provide a cost. They are the ones who burn up your phone lines and require a call center representative's assistance. But this cost is spread across the full 100% of your customers, so is not intolerable. Hidden profits and hidden costs = promotion and bonus.

Lest you say this scenario is far-fetched, I speak to these people. My colleagues at work speak to these people. What will happen is these unfortunates will call in, they will say something to the effect of, "I've been cancelled." or, "I signed up for COBRA but my insurance carrier never received my information." As a call center representative you can only dive in so far, but it soon becomes apparent that someone, somewhere, dropped the ball. People are apparently cancelled for no good reason whatsoever. One month they had coverage, the next, nothing.

And, these mistakes seem to go on for months. You will get a call from someone in August. It turns out they have been cancelled in March and they have never missed a payment. The way they found out about it was they tried to see a doctor in August only to find out they had no coverage dating back to March.

Someone had to process their payments and send them their bill. That's the COBRA administrator. They never get any indication there is a problem from them. Someone had to log their continuing status as insured with the insurance carrier. That's BDR.

Looking at some of these records, BDR apparently never received the information that this person took COBRA in the first place. So, in effect, every month the COBRA administrator collects the money and sends a data file to BDR. Every single month their billing side records that the person is current in their payments and that their coverage is continuing. Every single month that information fails to be transmitted to BDR.

But, with the vast majority of everyone else's information, their data seems to make the file fine every time.

This story leads me to a related tale of insurance payment chicanery. I spoke to a member living in my old home state of Montana. He is thinking of moving to a different state so he can get healthcare. "What?" You say. "Why can't he get healthcare in Montana?"

He does have retiree coverage through his employer. But, his insurer has been so slow to pay its doctors and hospitals in Montana that the area where he lives does not have a single doctor or hospital that is in their network. He would have to travel 60 to 100 miles for treatment by a network provider.

Believe me, this is a common occurrence in rural areas. I suspect it is an insurance company practice to stiff rural providers as a profit-generating strategy.

Why stiff rural people? Their sources of news and information are usually weak and so dependent on advertising dollars that they do not run critical exposés of any company. If there should happen to be a local crusading journalist, the damage is minimal as a rural area's low population limits the customer impact.

I'll write more about rural areas in the next section on retirement. Then, you'll have a good idea that your healthcare really sucks in rural America.

Retirement

You are set to retire. You have worked many long, hard years and now you look forward to some well earned rest.

Unfortunately, I am sad to have to break this to you, but this is where your healthcare truly sucks.

At my job, my calls get graded for quality. I recently lost some points for not congratulating a participant on their retirement.

I really don't feel like congratulating a person on their retirement. A baby, a marriage, a promotion, a raise, a job, a domestic partnership, these I can congratulate. But, a retirement, no.

Part of this is personal resentment. Most of the callers I work with have some type of pension benefits. These will provide some annuity income for the participants into their dotage.

I have no such benefits, in fact, BDR stopped contributing to my 401(k) at the beginning of 2009. So, I am truly on my own.

Let me ask you this question. Do you expect the pauper in the street to congratulate the wealthy burgher?

What gripes me about many of these pension benefits is they are for public utilities, government entities, or defense contractors. We have decided as a society that these people should receive a pension benefit as part of their compensation. Oftentimes, these benefits are under the scrutiny of a government panel, like a: public utility commission, county board of supervisors, or congressional committee. We figure that these workers, creating a public good, should have some compensation for their labor from their retirement unto their death.

I know that as I answer the calls of these participants; as I expend day after day of my precious labor, with little to no compensation directed to my retirement; as I take abuse from participants trying to collect their pension (I work with pension participants as well); as I am belittled, humiliated, insulted, and lampooned by insensitive angry participants; I know that I am helping to provide something that I will never have the chance to experience myself; I know that as my labor is being used to prop up the benefits of a previous generation that my own lack of retirement provision will result in a new burden to an upcoming cohort.

Besides, with what I know and what you will find out about retirement healthcare benefits, how can I in good conscience congratulate them?

Would you congratulate someone before their house burns down? Would you congratulate someone before they have to decide between food and healthcare?

Once again, lest you think I'm being hyperbolic, I speak to these participants. When your pension benefit is $2,000 per month and your retiree health coverage is $1,400, then you don't have much to fall back on for your immediate physical needs, like: food, clothing, and shelter.

One of my co-workers always talks about how he would quit his job with BDR if it weren't for his two bad habits, of eating regularly and wanting to have a roof over his head. I guess clothes aren't a concern. And, judging by his wardrobe, he is gaining full utilization of past purchases.

I guess what really burns me up about pensions is that I am expected to pay for so many others' pensions without benefit of my own. I pay for the county and city employees' pensions with my local taxes, the federal employees' and defense contractors' employees' with my federal income tax, oil workers' and utility workers' pensions with every fill-up and electric bill.

With the bailout of the automakers I am paying theirs, too, along with the bonuses of those Wall Street bankers. It is like being subjected to a candy tax. Every transaction has to pay the candy tax but I am not able to enjoy the candy.

I think of some waitress or other worker who has it even worse than myself. This person is constantly giving from their meagerness for the retirement safety of someone who is probably completing some job of comparable worth.

This discourse may not be so off-topic.

Most people with retiree health benefits have a pension. This gives the company something to deduct the cost of retiree health from. So, they really do go hand-in-hand.

But, getting back to healthcare. This is where the screwing really takes place. Especially, if you retire prior to age 65.

Why age 65? That is the age of your Medicare eligibility. Typically, Medicare policies cost less than the retiree policies up to age 65. As a pre-65 retiree, this is where you are going to take it in the shorts.

Oftentimes, on the phone, someone who is planning to retire prior to age 65 calls in. They want to know how much their retiree healthcare will cost.

After I give them the costs, frequently above $1,000 for a couple, they will be shocked. SHOCKED! That it is so much.

This will lead to a conversation of Why? I hate a conversation of Why?!

Why is it so expensive? Why so much? Why, that can't be right, can it? Why? (Insert John Lennon's scream of "Why?" from The Beatles "Revolution 9" here or for country fans, Johnny Cash's "Cry, Cry, Cry.")

As the benefits specialist that I am, I can only give mild descriptions of the rising cost of health coverage; how it increases as you get older, how group coverage works. These answers never seem to satisfy the why seeker.

Here, on this page, unencumbered by the need for politeness, I will give you the answers I always want to provide to the participants.

It is because you are old and you will get sick. You will cost the insurance company money. You may be able to get lower-cost individual coverage as an age 50 retiree but what about the cost of your individual coverage at age 64 when you've had a couple heart attacks. Then, a thousand dollars a month may seem cheap.

Sure, you can forego your group coverage now for the cheaper individual coverage of a 50-year-old but what about the future? Will your company or government allow you to return to group coverage? Or, have you sold your birthright for some pottage?

One government that I work for changed their retiree coverage a couple of years ago. Before that time their group coverage included both employees and retirees. Then, they switched to what is known as split-pool coverage.

Split-pool describes the splitting of employees and retirees into two groups. That way, the employees pay the group cost of coverage for employees and retirees for retirees. This particular government, let's call them Yellow County, is now being sued by its retirees.

The retirees are basically claiming that Yellow County is balancing its budget on the backs of the retirees. The retirees claim that the $10 million in savings the county is experiencing, is the result of shifting $10 million in costs to the retirees' premiums.

The retirees claim to have been part of a social contract wherein active employees would help pay retirees' rates in the knowledge that they would reap the same benefits on their retirement. This social contract having been broken by Yellow County on the splitting of their groups.

Yellow County recently introduced a premium holiday for its employees. Employees in the PPO plans will not have to pay premiums for six months as there are more than sufficient surpluses in these plans. Retirees are facing rate increases from 1-83% depending on their plan choice for 2010.

The perils of Yellow County retirees are not particular to government. Many of the private sector retirees I work with are facing the same rising costs and shrinking or slowly growing company contributions in the face of double-digit healthcare inflation.

Surprisingly, the retirees who catch the worst of this once were the higher-paid white-collar workers. These are the folks who were the most valuable during their work lives. They earned the highest amounts of pay, had the best benefits and perquisites.

The retirees who do the best tend to be union retirees, specifically, the retirees from unions that had the foresight to negotiate retiree health benefits for their workers. The current union workers then have incentive to fight for their own and the retirees' healthcare.

The white-collar retirees never had need of a union while they were working. Their wages climbed with the scarcity and desirability of their skills. Naively, many of them felt the company would look after them after they had outlived their usefulness.

These white-collar retirees are the ones the companies turn to for increased contributions. Because they never desired bargaining power while they worked, they have none now; and lack any leverage to get any. What is a retiree to do, go on strike?

In addition to retirees getting hosed by their former employers, rural America also takes it in the shorts. You would figure as a person who has devoted your life to a major corporation, often moving at their behest to a foreign location or enduring a big-city lifestyle, that your retirement years would be your own — you would think that you would be free to move to a location of your choosing when set free from the company's encumbrance. And, you are, technically. You can go where you want, but investigate before you move, as rural America may be financially off-limits.

Unsuspecting retirees would call me at BDR, having moved from California to Nevada. What could possibly change about their coverage? If your company is primarily based in one particular state, you may find it is the case that your retiree coverage changes drastically if you move to any other state. In many of these cases the increase could top $1,000 a month in premium difference.

Retirees in the know would call ahead, and often rule out the possibility of a move based primarily on the premium increase. This kind of post-job lock, differentiating it from the job lock that occurs during your work career when you can't quit a job for fear of losing your benefits, mitigates strongly against rural America.

Small towns all across the country would love to have these retirees. Their pensions and Social Security benefits would help provide stability of income and cause a growth of services for these folks.

Many of these small towns struggle as generation after generation of young people move to urban centers for greater opportunity. As these small towns attempt to attract retirees who could repopulate in their desire for a slower lifestyle, the cost of company retiree health coverage can present an insurmountable barrier. This, combined with the previously discussed inability to secure quality care in rural areas, is a serious hurdle that rural America is falling short of crossing. (Note: Since writing about how one rural area was essentially being boycotted by an insurer, I have read more and it seems the local hospital administration may be to blame for suspect billing practices. I wanted to share this as an example of the complexities involved. The result remains that this person cannot get health service from his local hospital as they no longer accept his insurance.)

———————————

You are getting ready to turn age 65. You have been looking forward to this since you retired. You figure that with Medicare beginning you are going to see a serious drop in your health premiums.

You are happy to know that Medicare is going to be there for you. You've paid in all these years and you are looking for some payback.

You know there is a prescription drug benefit and you've heard of Medicare Advantage or Senior HMO's. Ultimately, you figure this will be the last major health insurance decision you will have to make.

———————————

Permit me to divert course from Medicare for a moment. I have a correction. "Revolution 9" by The Beatles does not seem to have someone screaming "Why?" I listened to it A LOT. Most of my listening took place on September 9, 2009 — 9/9/9 by strange coincidence. It does seem to contain John Lennon screaming "Right". This sounds very close to "Why" but it is not, indeed, "Why". The song also contains the line, "Every year he got another year older and another year slower." As I just had a birthday, I can relate. At 44, I am halfway between my college graduation and Medicare.

At 23, I felt pretty invincible; at 44 I am still doing well despite my mystery ailment. Who knows what 65 will bring?

Permit me another diversion in my discourse. My old senator Max Baucus released his version of healthcare reform this week. In the interest of disclosure, let me say that I like Senator Baucus. I'm from Montana and it being a state of small population, eventually you have dealings with just about everybody, or their friend.

I used to own Senator Baucus' father's car. The Green Dragon was a 1974 Dodge Monaco Brougham station wagon. I loved that car. Before I sold it I asked the Senator if he had wanted it. Apparently, it had been a deathbed request of his father that he have the car.

Senator Baucus sent me a nice note on official Senate stationery thanking me for the offer. As much as I like Senator Baucus, I do not think his reform measure touches on the subject of this book which is the administration of your healthcare. It leaves the current state of administration as it is.

In my personal life I am just now getting over a bout with what I assume was the flu. It was undiagnosed as I never saw a doctor, but I had a high fever and basically stayed home and slept a lot. Luckily, I do have sick days I can use from my work. I missed an entire week. Some of this was to avoid infecting others, but really I was in no shape to work during that time. Even now, I feel like I have a little bit of it, but time to plunge back into the public swim.

Much has been made of how the Baucus plan does not call for negotiation of prescription drug prices for Medicare Part D patients. The U.S. Government does negotiate prescription drug prices for the Veterans Health Administration. Virtually every other government in the world negotiates prescription prices. But, the non-negotiation of drug prices will continue for the Medicare Part D benefit.

I don't believe a negotiation exists when one of the parties refuses to negotiate. This would leave the pharmaceutical industry to set its own prices, the U.S. Gov't to pay them through its subsidies of the Medicare Part D prescription drug benefit. As a general principle, I think there ought to be some consensus that the U.S. Gov't should fulfill its fiduciary responsibility by negotiating drug prices. I don't know why this reasonable assumption should not be part of reform.

I have heard and read that the White House and Senator Baucus crafted as part of the healthcare reform deal a promise not to negotiate drug prices. All right, suppose I accept that. What is the pharmaceutical part of the deal? What do they have to give? This I have not heard, but I suppose that they may have agreed to not block healthcare reform legislation.

This has gone far afield from where we were talking about Medicare, but it goes to show what a political football your healthcare becomes when it transitions to the realm of Medicare. Decisions made at the highest levels in Washington will now affect your healthcare.

In the time of my break of writing this, I have heard that the pharmaceutical part of the supposed deal is X number of billions of dollars that Big Pharma will contribute to lower the cost of medications as part of healthcare reform. This is a backdoor negotiation that simply demonstrates my argument about the need for government negotiation of drug prices. The drug manufacturers apparently just don't want it enshrined into law.

In other words, "Trust us... to deliver

on the billions of savings. If they don't appear....well, it's not like it's illegal. So, what are you gonna do about it? Huh? Huh? What? What are you gonna do about it? "

Recently, they have been announcing the Nobel prizes. One fellow who won it for physics was speaking about his retirement. He retired at age 55 in the 1980's and spent 17 years sailing about the globe. He must have had a great pension and health scheme.

However, if you are just a middling technocrat you are subject to the vagaries of your employer and the whimsy of the market and maybe you'll have a retirement and retiree health and maybe not. It reminds me of a story of a scientist who actually made an important discovery. Apparently, he did not capitalize on it. He was, not too recently, driving an airport-shuttle bus.

Let's take the bus back to the scene of your Medicare retirement. We'll start with the basics. Most folks will be able to get Medicare A at no cost. Medicare A covers bills from hospitalization.

However, some public-sector employees have never had their employer (a local government) pay in for Medicare A coverage. When they retire they would have to either pay a premium for Medicare A or get coverage to pay for the uncovered hospitalization. The local government I work with has plans that cover this deficit. So, not much of a problem.

Medicare Part B requires a premium that is currently $96.40 for most participants. Some of the lusher participants have a higher premium and some of the lower-income folks are subsidized. Medicare B covers doctor visits. Most people have it deducted from their Social Security payments.

Toss into this mix the plans known as Medicare Advantage or Senior HMO's. Typically, Medicare is your primary coverage and your employer may provide what would be called supplemental or secondary coverage. A Medicare Advantage plan actually takes the place of Medicare.

Let me provide an example that may help to explain the difference. Under regular Medicare you get a doctor's bill for $100. Medicare typically pays 80%. So, Medicare would pay $80. Then your supplemental coverage would catch the rest. After you had met a deductible, your plan might pay 80%. So, your plan would pay 80% of the $20 that is left. Your plan would pay $16 and you would pay $4.

Under Medicare Advantage you

actually assign your Medicare to an HMO. This requires an enrollment form and an enrollment process. Then, when you visit your physician you would only have to pay a co-pay.

I imagine the original selling point of Medicare Advantage was that this type of program would save money. It turns out it does. But, the HMO's who are saving this money do not want to have their reimbursements cut.

One recent government study said that Medicare Advantage plans were receiving 14% more than the cost of the coverage provided to seniors. This provides a tidy profit.

In a perverse display of economic wisdom. Congress, I think it was Republican-controlled at the time, wanted to cut Medicare reimbursement rates to doctors. This was for the typical Medicare scheme. Medicare Advantage was to have no such cut. As I remember it, Congress was trying to have the doctor's reimbursement cut by about 14%.

So, in other words, Congress was trying to cut the efficient doctor's rates by 14% and keep the inefficient HMO's rates inflated by 14%. I can imagine someone arguing the opposite side of this. Here is their argument.

"Medicare Advantage HMO's are efficient and seniors get additional services like vision and dental, etc. Traditional Medicare is inefficient and should have cuts because it is getting increasingly expensive."

I guess I would argue back that if Medicare Advantage can provide additional services for 14% less then we should enjoy the cost savings. Also, it is tough for these Medicare patients to find doctors who accept Medicare. The reimbursement rates for regular patients are oftentimes regarded as insufficient.

In addition, Medicare Advantage plans have an incentive to sign up the youngest, healthiest seniors. They do this partly through "teaser" rates when they first become Medicare eligible. This might be the come-on; that Medicare Advantage would require no additional premium beyond that you would pay for Medicare B. They never inform you that it may increase as you get older.

If you are getting confused by the arguments I am making and the information I am providing to you, imagine how a 65-, 75-, or 85-year-old feels. Part of the beauty of Medicare is its simplicity. You sign up a few months before your 65th birthday. Then, it is in place for the rest of your life, barring missing premiums. Since the premiums are coming from your Social Security check, this is mostly unlikely.

The confuseopoly (thanks, Scott Adams) created by Medicare Advantage is compounded by the administrative headache of actually getting a person signed up for Medicare Advantage. Because this person is actually assigning their Medicare benefits to an insurer, they need to go through an enrollment process.

Let me describe how this works in an ideal example. You call your benefits center to sign up for a Medicare Advantage plan. Because you are calling at least two months in advance, we have plenty of time to sign you up for a Medicare Advantage plan.

In the confirmation statement of your benefit election you will receive an enrollment form. This form will need to be filled out and either returned to the HMO or your benefits administrator, depending.

This enrollment form is then processed and when the person becomes Medicare Advantage-eligible they slide right into the Medicare Advantage HMO. Obviously, in real life, we deal with un-ideal situations.

Permit me to interrupt this completely uninteresting example of Medicare Advantage to tell of a phone call at work. This fella calls in and tells his sad story of claims denied for coordination of benefits[*] issues.

This guy had had his spouse on his coverage and everytime the spouse had to go to the doctor or the hospital they used his insurance. Every. Single. Time. In the thousands of dollars the bills were. This went on for five years. How many times do *you* visit the doctor in five years?

Anyway, at the end of the five years I think he had a major expense for his spouse. I think she went to the hospital or something to that effect. Well, this triggered the man's insurance to do some investigating. They discovered that the spouse had her own retiree coverage.

This discovery, then, allowed them to disallow all five years of claims as they were not the primary insurer for the spouse. The insurance company considered themselves the secondary coverage so they basically said all five years of claims payment were voided.

---

[*] Coordination of benefits refers to which insurer will pay first, or be primary, and which will pay next, or secondary.

So, now, the guy, he has five years worth of unpaid claims. Well, when he goes to the spouse's insurer, they say they will only allow claims to be submitted within one year of service.

So, this guy has to eat four years worth of claims. As a call center representative, you become kind of inured to these tales of woe. It seems like every day you hear of a new story of a new indignity a fellow human being is forced to endure in their search for quality healthcare.

Some of the more sensitive souls simply do not make it in this job. People who see the utter ridiculosity in shuffling electrons to and fro, to prevent payment, deny service, pass the buck.

One of my favorite heroes was the call center representative who hung up on a member as he was in full-throated call trying to get his healthcare in place. The representative hung up and walked out of the call center, forever. The last words he uttered were something like, "This job is going to give me a heart attack or a stroke."

I can relate to this sensitive soul. Perhaps, you could tell having read this far. But, unlike him, I have a higher tolerance for the suffering of others.

Let's get back to Medicare Advantage. God, I know it's dull, but here goes. I just gave you the ideal Medicare Advantage scenario. The diligent participant fills in their paperwork and sends it in on time and everyone is happy. Now, let's get back to the real world.

The real participant may or may not even realize they are becoming Medicare-eligible at age 65. (If you think this is unrealistic, let me tell you of a call I with a doctor. A DOCTOR. He seemingly had no knowledge of the workings of Medicare. None. He did not seem to realize he became Medicare-eligible at age 65.) Let's figure our example has a little more on the ball than that. Our participant actually signs up for Medicare. But, this participant does not make his elections with the benefits center.

When a Medicare-eligible participant fails to make an election in time, they may be put into what is known as default coverage. Let's say they become Medicare-eligible on Nov. 1st, 2010.

The participant gets put into his default coverage on Nov. 1st. But, let's say the participant comes to and realizes he needs to make some sort of decision. He decides he wants a futzing Medicare Advantage plan.

Now, the participant has to go through the whole enrollment process for Medicare Advantage. He has to fill out an enrollment form. He's got to send that in and await approval from Medicare for his entry. In the meantime, he is cooling his heels in the default coverage.

Let me give you an example of the mess this can cause. The participant is cruising along pre-65 in HMO X. The participant gets defaulted into a PPO plan on Nov. 1st with his entry into Medicare. This default election generates a confirmation that is sent to the participant.

When he receives the confirmation he realizes his mistake and calls in to us at the benefits center. If this participant had some medical care scheduled for the first two weeks of November with HMO X, when HMO X learns that you don't have their coverage they will be denying your claims. Because you just entered PPO Y you will have to meet their deductible before your co-insurance kicks in.

You could be out $300, $500, or more. Then, you may have the exact same situation on the side of your prescription coverage. If you had any prescriptions filled you may have to meet a new separate prescription deductible.

You are becoming Medicare-eligible. You have heard there is a new prescription benefit. You think that sounds good. You figure you could use some help with your prescription drug costs.

In talking to your benefits specialist you understand that you will be getting a prescription drug benefit with your employer-provided retiree health coverage.

On to Medicare Part D or the prescription drug benefit through Medicare. When this was being created, Congress did not want to have all the employer coverages jettison their prescription drug benefits. I believe they created a subsidy for existing plans. In signing up for your employer-based retiree coverage, Medicare wants to prevent fraud and double-dipping for prescription benefits.

This was a big problem in the first year of Medicare Part D. People were getting signed up for multiple plans. Some safeguards had to be put into place. Now, if you sign up for another drug benefit or even another medical plan with a prescription drug benefit, your employer-based coverage will be cancelled. You get a chance to return, still, it is a major hassle.

That friendly-looking man at the mall that is talking you grandmother into low-cost drugs. He is after that sweet commission. If it messes up granny's heart medication, he's on to the next senior.

The above paragraph may sound exceedingly cynical. But, I am one of the people you are going to have to call to get this mess straightened out. So, I am tired of cleaning up after insurance salesmen.

What breaks my heart is the senior who is obviously confused and should be getting some help from a son or daughter, friend or neighbor. They call me and I have to sort out what I consider to be a completely unnecessary snafu.

Medicare used to be a very simple program. You signed up once when you turned 65. Then, you really did not have to think about it until you died. Now, with Medicare Advantage and the Medicare Part D prescription drug benefit, you have to make a decision virtually every single year and you are constantly being confronted with traps and pitfalls.

Where is the sense in this? Why take our most vulnerable, infirm, and addled population and subject them to unscrupulous salespeople, hidden costs, denials of service, refusals of prescriptions, unnecessary paperwork, confusing terms, and a general lack of dignity and sympathy.

Does this make sense to anyone?

Up to this point I have painted a bleak portrait of my job and co-workers. We are the folks who have to say "No" and enforce the plan rules. Sometimes that means telling your grandmother that she is simply going to have to find a way on her fixed income to pay out-of-pocket for her heart medicine. Then, once the mess of her prescription drug benefit is sorted out she can submit a claim for reimbursement.

However, my co-workers and myself can be your best friends and allies when there is an emergency or we have the power to resolve your dilemma. You see, we know about these traps and gotchas. We know how to get your coverage reinstated.

In a true emergency we can really hustle and make sure your husband who was in a car accident gets admitted to the hospital. These moments can be satisfying. Helping someone, making sure they have the care they need, these times make it all worthwhile.

And, hopefully you have more than a few positive moments every day when you do help someone with their benefits. It helps to remember that we are trying to take care of people's healthcare needs.

One common quality of the call center representatives I work with, the ones who stick around anyway, is that we do care about assisting people. We are in customer service because we truly want to help you with your problems, despite how frustrating you can be at times.

(And, on a side note, I think call center representatives and customer service folks can make some of the most annoying callers and customers. This includes myself. When we get terrible service, we know how good service should be done so we tell you. In fact, I think we go a little overboard at times, myself included.

Also, having to be unfailingly polite to someone on the other end of a phone line takes a psychic toll. All that suppressed rage has to come out on someone. Sorry, other customer service folks.

I wrote a poem of the spiritual aspects of call center work. Allow me to share it here.

For a Call Center Representative

Can I be official
  without being officious?
Can I be glad
 without being glib?
Let me be serious
 without being sedate.
Let me be fast
 without being frenzied.
Let me be calm
 without being callous.
Please let me say
  what needs to be said
 without saying more
    or being a bore.
Let me be myself
 without being robotic
And show my personality
without seeming neurotic.
Finally, Please let me care
 And respect everyone's
    fundamental humanity;
   No matter who they are,
  Or, who they know,
  Or, what they say,
  Or, how they sound,
 Even if I want to reach
    through the phone cord
   Grab their tongue,
   And, strangle them.
   Even if.

_____

87

In trying to see everyone's importance and worth, I think I have grown as a person.)

I was going to save the sales pitch for last but feel that I need to go ahead and insert it here. It seems appropriate.

Sales Pitch

I am an advocate of single-payer healthcare reform. So many of the items I have complained about would simply not exist with a single-payer system.

When you were born you would be signed up for a medical plan much like you get a Social Security number. Since Medicare basically uses your SSN anyway, why not just have one Social Security/Medical Security number?

That's essentially it. No more electron shuffling. Virtually every problem I have addressed in *Your Healthcare Sucks*, would vanish or be transmuted to a new, different, and simpler problem. We'll always have problems. (Thanks, Desmond Dekker.)

I won't go back over everything. I'll leave that up to you. In some ways this book has been a mystery with a single elegant solution at its end.

One thing that would be a significant change would be my job. Most of the health and welfare tasks would simply not exist. You've heard me describe my job, would that be such a bad thing?

Perhaps, I would have to get a different job. I don't think I would ever make it as a salesman. What do you think?

Death

You'd think death would be the end of your healthcare suckiness. In reality, it continues.

Often, an employer plan will offer coverage to a surviving spouse. Typically, this is for retirees only. If you die as an employee, your surviving spouse is not entitled to any healthcare benefits. With the exception being if you were retirement eligible.

With a domestic partner on your coverage, someone to whom you are not legally married, that person would not be considered a surviving spouse, so would have no further healthcare benefits. Your benefits end with your death. Sorry, gay couples and shacker-uppers.

These folks may even have a hard time qualifying for COBRA. COBRA is a federal benefit, after all. So, rules of morality and virtue don't require the non-wed to have a coverage extension. Some employers step into the breach here and do offer COBRA to domestic partners.

You are a surviving spouse and enjoy being safe in the knowledge your employer-based healthcare benefits will continue.

But, you have happened to find love at an advanced age. You are thinking of getting married but wonder how it will affect your benefits.

You are very right to wonder. In fact, you may want to give a quick call to your benefits administrator before you put a ring on it. (Thanks, Beyoncé.)

With some employers, simply getting married will cause your surviving spouse coverage to terminate. With others, it is the act of trying to add your new spouse as a dependent that will cause your coverage to be cancelled. Just don't ever try to add your spouse as a dependent and you'll be fine.

In the first instance, you may want to remain single for the health benefits, much as some seniors remain single for the tax benefits. It is cheaper to file single than married, I believe.

In the time I have been writing this book, my company, BDR, has become the takeover target of a large copier concern, Zifuz. We've been assured there won't be any changes to our jobs but the fear of more layoffs and reduced circumstances looms.

The CEO of BDR has an interesting hobby of photographing the homeless. He gives them each a twenty-dollar bill. He has been the subject of a television piece and has gallery shows.

This activity causes mixed feelings. You can see it as exploitive, artistic, humanitarian, self-aggrandizing.

I was speaking with a BDR call center representative about it. Her reaction to the amount paid to the people, which also encapsulates all those mixed feelings, was, "That's all?"

Afterword - About the Author

I learned about single-payer healthcare at my first non-factory job out of college with the Montana Senior Citizens Association (MSCA). This was back in 1991 in Helena, Montana.

The MSCA had just had a resolution passed through the Montana legislature advocating a single-payer healthcare system. Yes, 1991.

The good folks of MSCA helped convince me of the superiority of a single-payer healthcare system. Granted, I really didn't know a lot about the issue when I started. But, I have never failed to see the logic since.

I know there are many and serious opponents of single-payer. There are even some friends who won't give us a hearing, Senator Max Baucus. Ironically, it was he who wrote up the incorporation papers for MSCA at its founding when he was a young, idealistic lawyer.

Not to belittle but to simplify their arguments I would put them in two camps. First, no one supports single-payer. This is along the lines of self-fulfilling prophecy. If I never ask the question, "Who wants candy?" so no one ever answers that they want candy...therefore, no one wants candy. It is simply the ostrich effect. Ignore virtually the rest of the industrial nations and they seemingly go away.

Secondly, the government can't run anything right. For people who believe this, I have a challenge. If you don't think single-payer would be popular and efficient, try to convince any senior to give up their Medicare.

Addendum A

Today I work in a Potemkin village. No Internet surfing (my chosen vice), cell phones, music listening, portable digital devices are in sight. Banners have been hung from the ceiling with care in hopes that a major passenger railroad will purchase our services.

We had another potential client on-site earlier this week. At that time motivational corporate posters sprung up on our walls. Mostly they have now been framed and are mounted on the wall.

A lady from the railroad walked by. She saw me looking for the weather for the championship game between the Grizzlies and the Wildcats. She and her teammates were dressed in identical terry cloth shirts of blue like a bowling team or a cult.

That Internet is hard to resist. And, for someone like myself who is prone to flights of imagination and a desire to learn a specific piece of information immediately, it is an almost irresistible temptation.

There are a couple of things I wanted to add to the fact that your healthcare sucks. I'm not sure I emphasized how stupid it is to have the IRS as the major governmental administrator of healthcare law. Or, do I really need to point that out.

Also, I think I missed informing you of the perverse incentive that companies have to drop retiree coverage. The worse retiree coverage is, the more expensive, the greater the deductibles and co-pays, the more likely retirees will drop their coverage through the company. This is a boon to the firm as this will lower their overall retiree healthcare burden. This is a bust for the remaining retirees as they will then see the coverage costs increase because there will be fewer retirees to carry the burden of the group, thus, leading to more retirees dropping coverage.

This, combined with a change at the corporate level from open-ended retiree healthcare commitments to dollar-amount specific commitments practically guarantees a worsening of the retiree healthcare environment. Let me provide an example.

Company X has a commitment stated in its documents or summary plan description to provide 80% of retiree healthcare costs. As double-digit insurance inflation compounded through the last several years, company X discovered it was pouring forth more and more money for retiree healthcare, a non-revenue producing item.

Offering to pay for a certain percentage of a cost is an open-ended commitment. For example, 80% of $100 is $80, 80% of $1000 is $800. You can see how this might drive company accountants mad. How can you predict future healthcare costs when you have no control over insurance rates?

So, company X decides to change its commitment to retiree healthcare costs to a closed-end dollar amount. Company X decides to limit their maximum retiree burden to $500 per retiree.

Oftentimes, a remnant of their previous distribution remains. For example, some companies had employee's years of service reflected as a percentage of the company's contribution. After 30 years of service you would be entitled to 100% of the company contribution.

When the company commitment was open-ended you would get 100% of the 80%

of the cost of retiree health coverage. If the insurance costs $1,000 a month, you would get 100% of the 80% of the $1,000 or $800.

With the change to a closed-end dollar commitment the retiree would get 100% of the dollar amount, in this case $500. Simple enough, right.

Addendum B

My aim has been to explore healthcare administration. In other words, how you and your family get access to healthcare through your employer.

Even as I write these words the prevalence of employer-based coverage is diminishing. Between 2008 and 2009 the percentage of people covered by employment-based health insurance decreased from 58.5% to 55.8%, the lowest since recording began in 1987.[1]

While the number of people covered

---

[1] U.S. Department of Commerce, Economics and Statistics Administration, U.S. Census Bureau. Income, Poverty, and Health Insurance Coverage in the United States: 2009. Carmen DeNavas-Walt, Bernadette D. Proctor, Jessica C. Smith. issued September 2010

through their employers fall, there are forces trying to turn back the tide, notably, the Patient Protection and Affordable Care Act. This is known by my Republican callers as "Obamacare", almost always said with menace. As for the representatives, we refer to it as "Puhpaca" or "Pea-Packa'" or we spell it out as "P-P-A-C-A".

There have been some small gains with subsidies to small employers to have them provide coverage. I doubt this will stop the slide.

There are four major portions of the law and these are subject to the same forces that are rending healthcare today. If anything, the law will either slow the collapse or speed the disintegration. It is tough to determine. The outcome does not seem in question to me. The ultimate result will have to be something akin to single-payer or one of the other methods hit upon by the industrial nations of the world.

These four sections are:

1. Individual mandate.
2. Subsidies.
3. Insurance pools.
4. Regulation of insurers to maintain payout targets.

The individual mandate is unlikely to be successful. The authors of the law realized this and thus added subsidies so that individuals could buy into the system. Even a modest effort in this direction was less successful than planned.

As part of the American Recovery and Reinvestment Act (the popularly named "Stimulus Package"), a subsidy was provided to assist formerly-employed workers afford COBRA coverage. This act, although predicted to have helped seven million people, actually appears to have helped far fewer. "This finding has implications for the impact of the subsidies that will become available in 2014 under provisions of the Patient and Protection and Affordable Care Act of 2010 (P.L. 111-148), the heath reform law known as PPACA. Those subsidies may not have as large an effect as predicted when PPACA was passed. As a result, the number of uninsured may not fall as much as predicted."[2]

Health insurance pools have been used largely unsuccessfully at the state level for years. This is simply taking a failed idea and making it larger.

---

[2] Paul Fonstin. EBRI Employee Benefit Research Institute Notes, Vol. 31, No. 10, (October 2010): 14, Employee Benefit Research Institute.

Finally, the regulation of insurers, to hold them to particular rates of payout, is supposed to impede the increasing climb of health premiums. The insurers get some additional customers through the individual mandate and the subsidies. They, in turn, have to submit to the government's oversight.

Here, I will appeal to the reader's opinion of insurers' trustworthiness. Substitute brokerages or banks for insurers and the conflicts of interest become apparent. Insurers will always want to maximize profit, or their reserves, in the case of non-profits. Their track record has not been the most confidence-inspiring.

True, Germany and Switzerland have relied on private insurers to provide coverage with success. Time will tell if the United States can make the same gamble and win. The reader may have guessed where I am putting my money.

———

You are looking forward to adding your dependent child who is no longer a full-time student but who is still under age 26.

You know there has been a change as a result of healthcare reform and it makes you happy to be able to add your dependent child.

You just aren't sure about how to do it.

━━━━━━━━━━━━━━━━━━━━━━━━

So far, the only real change healthcare reform has wrought for administration has been in the area of full-time student coverage. Basically, you can keep a dependent child on your coverage until age 26 as long as they are not eligible for coverage through an employer.

On the surface, you may be thinking, "great", but if you looked a little deeper you may come to the realization that one petty bureaucratic requirement has been substituted for another.

Also, all of the problems and dilemmas of the full-time student process have their corollaries in the new regulation. For example, what is "employed"? Is it full-time, part-time, seasonal, etc.? What is considered being eligible through your employer? Is it just enough to be offered something, even if you can't afford it? What if the policy is crap? Is there a medium threshold of quality?

These are just the questions off the top of my head. And, of course, there are no good answers for any of these. I'm back to nudging and fluffing these participants off the phone. Parents whose children are denied coverage for failing one of these tests may have differing ideas of what constitutes employment and coverage.

It is one more hoop to jump through, and, as if I have to remind you of Montgomery's Axiom, some will fail.

A few months back I spoke to a new mom whose child had been in desperate trouble from birth. She had racked up over a quarter-million dollars in charges. Well, this mom had been so busy, that she forgot to add the child during the 30-day window. She said she had talked to everybody who assured her the child had been added. She, though, never called her benefits administrator.

I wrote her name down so I could keep track of her appeal. I think I lost this note.

Now, I can't remember her name.

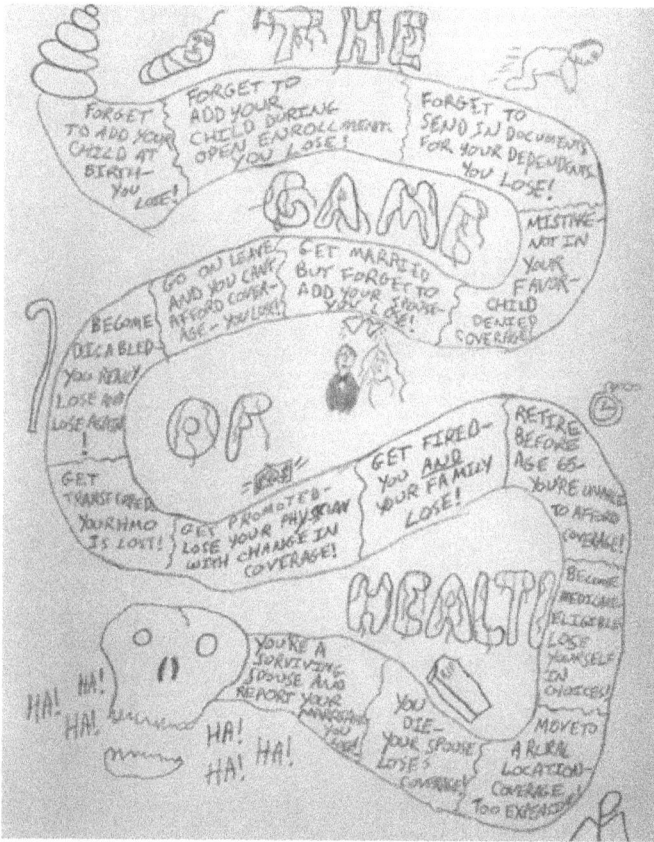

Other Works by the Author

Lies

Lies '99
(Rocket e-book)

Party Like a Lacrosse Star

Coming Soon from Googolplex Publishing

The Outrider: Collected Columns 2000-2006

Lies
(21st Century Edition)

www.ingramcontent.com/pod-product-compliance
Lightning Source LLC
Chambersburg PA
CBHW031216270326
41931CB00006B/577